GRATITUDE WEEKLY PLANNER

Week of: _____

GRATITUDE goals

TO-DO

	Monday	Tuesday	Wednesday	Thursday	Friday	Saturday	Sunday
ACTIVITIES							
FOCUS							
GRATITUDE							

REFLECTIONS

EXCITED FOR	POSITIVE THOUGHT	KINDNESS

NOTES

GRATITUDE WEEKLY PLANNER

Week of: _____

GRATITUDE goals

TO-DO

	Monday	Tuesday	Wednesday	Thursday	Friday	Saturday	Sunday
ACTIVITIES							
FOCUS							
GRATITUDE							

REFLECTIONS

EXCITED FOR	POSITIVE THOUGHT	KINDNESS

NOTES

GRATITUDE WEEKLY PLANNER

Week of: _____

GRATITUDE goals

TO-DO

	Monday	Tuesday	Wednesday	Thursday	Friday	Saturday	Sunday
ACTIVITIES							
FOCUS							
GRATITUDE							

REFLECTIONS

EXCITED FOR	POSITIVE THOUGHT	KINDNESS

NOTES

GRATITUDE WEEKLY PLANNER

Week of: _____

GRATITUDE *goals*

_____
_____
_____
_____
_____
_____

TO-DO

_____
_____
_____
_____
_____
_____

	Monday	Tuesday	Wednesday	Thursday	Friday	Saturday	Sunday
ACTIVITIES							
FOCUS							
GRATITUDE							

REFLECTIONS

EXCITED FOR	POSITIVE THOUGHT	KINDNESS

NOTES

_____
_____
_____
_____
_____

GRATITUDE WEEKLY PLANNER

Week of: _____

GRATITUDE goals

TO-DO

Monday	Tuesday	Wednesday	Thursday	Friday	Saturday	Sunday

ACTIVITIES

FOCUS

GRATITUDE

REFLECTIONS

EXCITED FOR | POSITIVE THOUGHT | KINDNESS

NOTES

GRATITUDE WEEKLY PLANNER

Week of: _____

GRATITUDE goals

TO-DO

	Monday	Tuesday	Wednesday	Thursday	Friday	Saturday	Sunday
ACTIVITIES							
FOCUS							
GRATITUDE							

REFLECTIONS

EXCITED FOR	POSITIVE THOUGHT	KINDNESS

NOTES

GRATITUDE WEEKLY PLANNER

Week of: _____

GRATITUDE goals

_____
_____
_____
_____
_____
_____

TO-DO

_____
_____
_____
_____
_____
_____

	Monday	*Tuesday*	*Wednesday*	*Thursday*	*Friday*	*Saturday*	*Sunday*
ACTIVITIES							
FOCUS							
GRATITUDE							

REFLECTIONS

EXCITED FOR	POSITIVE THOUGHT	KINDNESS

NOTES

_____
_____
_____
_____
_____

GRATITUDE WEEKLY PLANNER

Week of: _____

GRATITUDE
goals

_____

_____

_____

_____

TO-DO

_____

_____

_____

_____

_____

_____

	Monday	Tuesday	Wednesday	Thursday	Friday	Saturday	Sunday
ACTIVITIES							
FOCUS							
GRATITUDE							

REFLECTIONS

EXCITED FOR	POSITIVE THOUGHT	KINDNESS

NOTES

_____

_____

_____

_____

_____

GRATITUDE WEEKLY PLANNER

Week of: _____

GRATITUDE goals

TO-DO

	Monday	Tuesday	Wednesday	Thursday	Friday	Saturday	Sunday
ACTIVITIES							
FOCUS							
GRATITUDE							

REFLECTIONS

EXCITED FOR	POSITIVE THOUGHT	KINDNESS

NOTES

GRATITUDE WEEKLY PLANNER

Week of: _____

GRATITUDE goals

TO-DO

	Monday	Tuesday	Wednesday	Thursday	Friday	Saturday	Sunday
ACTIVITIES							
FOCUS							
GRATITUDE							

REFLECTIONS

EXCITED FOR	POSITIVE THOUGHT	KINDNESS

NOTES

GRATITUDE WEEKLY PLANNER

Week of: _____

GRATITUDE goals

_____
_____
_____
_____
_____
_____

TO-DO

_____
_____
_____
_____
_____
_____

	Monday	Tuesday	Wednesday	Thursday	Friday	Saturday	Sunday
ACTIVITIES							
FOCUS							
GRATITUDE							

REFLECTIONS

EXCITED FOR	POSITIVE THOUGHT	KINDNESS

NOTES

_____
_____
_____
_____
_____

GRATITUDE WEEKLY PLANNER

Week of: _____

GRATITUDE *goals*

_____
_____
_____
_____
_____

TO-DO

_____
_____
_____
_____
_____
_____
_____

	Monday	Tuesday	Wednesday	Thursday	Friday	Saturday	Sunday
ACTIVITIES							
FOCUS							
GRATITUDE							

REFLECTIONS

EXCITED FOR	POSITIVE THOUGHT	KINDNESS

NOTES

_____
_____
_____
_____

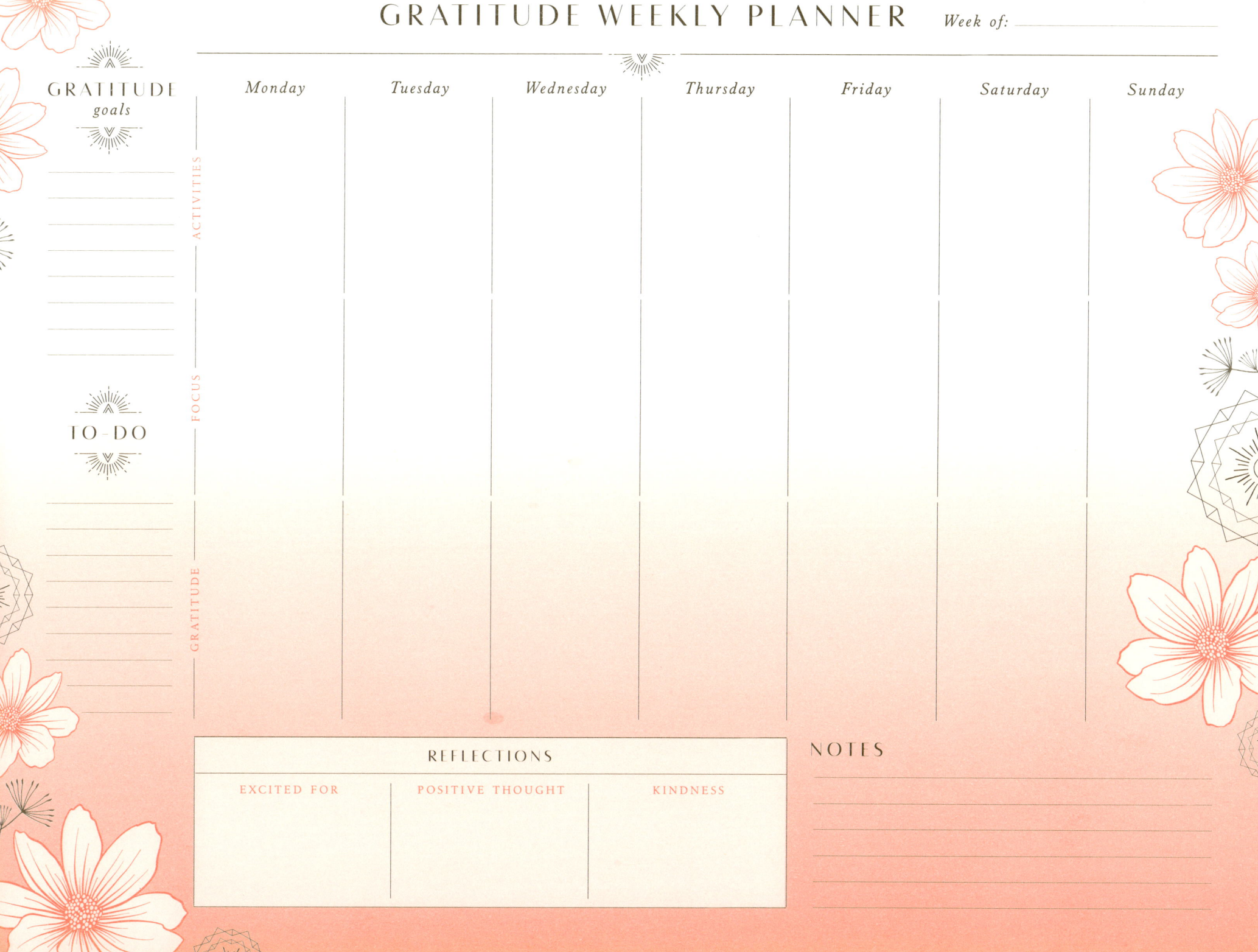

GRATITUDE WEEKLY PLANNER

Week of: _____

GRATITUDE goals

_____
_____
_____
_____
_____

TO-DO

_____
_____
_____
_____
_____
_____

	Monday	Tuesday	Wednesday	Thursday	Friday	Saturday	Sunday
ACTIVITIES							
FOCUS							
GRATITUDE							

REFLECTIONS

EXCITED FOR	POSITIVE THOUGHT	KINDNESS

NOTES

_____
_____
_____
_____
_____

GRATITUDE WEEKLY PLANNER

Week of: _____

GRATITUDE *goals*

TO-DO

	Monday	Tuesday	Wednesday	Thursday	Friday	Saturday	Sunday
ACTIVITIES							
FOCUS							
GRATITUDE							

REFLECTIONS

EXCITED FOR	POSITIVE THOUGHT	KINDNESS

NOTES

GRATITUDE WEEKLY PLANNER

Week of: _____

GRATITUDE goals

_____
_____
_____
_____
_____

TO-DO

_____
_____
_____
_____
_____
_____

	Monday	*Tuesday*	*Wednesday*	*Thursday*	*Friday*	*Saturday*	*Sunday*
ACTIVITIES							
FOCUS							
GRATITUDE							

REFLECTIONS

EXCITED FOR	POSITIVE THOUGHT	KINDNESS

NOTES

_____
_____
_____
_____
_____

GRATITUDE WEEKLY PLANNER

Week of: _____

GRATITUDE goals

_____
_____
_____
_____
_____

TO-DO

_____
_____
_____
_____
_____
_____

	Monday	Tuesday	Wednesday	Thursday	Friday	Saturday	Sunday
ACTIVITIES							
FOCUS							
GRATITUDE							

REFLECTIONS

EXCITED FOR	POSITIVE THOUGHT	KINDNESS

NOTES

_____
_____
_____
_____
_____

GRATITUDE WEEKLY PLANNER

Week of: _____

GRATITUDE goals

_____
_____
_____
_____
_____
_____

TO-DO

_____
_____
_____
_____
_____
_____

	Monday	Tuesday	Wednesday	Thursday	Friday	Saturday	Sunday
ACTIVITIES							
FOCUS							
GRATITUDE							

REFLECTIONS

EXCITED FOR	POSITIVE THOUGHT	KINDNESS

NOTES

_____
_____
_____
_____
_____

GRATITUDE WEEKLY PLANNER

Week of: _____

GRATITUDE *goals*

TO-DO

Monday	Tuesday	Wednesday	Thursday	Friday	Saturday	Sunday

ACTIVITIES

FOCUS

GRATITUDE

REFLECTIONS

EXCITED FOR | **POSITIVE THOUGHT** | **KINDNESS**

NOTES

GRATITUDE WEEKLY PLANNER

Week of: _____

GRATITUDE goals

TO-DO

	Monday	Tuesday	Wednesday	Thursday	Friday	Saturday	Sunday
ACTIVITIES							
FOCUS							
GRATITUDE							

REFLECTIONS

EXCITED FOR	POSITIVE THOUGHT	KINDNESS

NOTES

GRATITUDE WEEKLY PLANNER

Week of: _____

GRATITUDE goals

_____
_____
_____
_____
_____
_____

TO-DO

_____
_____
_____
_____
_____
_____

	Monday	Tuesday	Wednesday	Thursday	Friday	Saturday	Sunday
ACTIVITIES							
FOCUS							
GRATITUDE							

REFLECTIONS

EXCITED FOR	POSITIVE THOUGHT	KINDNESS

NOTES

_____
_____
_____
_____
_____

GRATITUDE WEEKLY PLANNER

Week of: _____

GRATITUDE goals

TO-DO

	Monday	Tuesday	Wednesday	Thursday	Friday	Saturday	Sunday
ACTIVITIES							
FOCUS							
GRATITUDE							

REFLECTIONS

EXCITED FOR	POSITIVE THOUGHT	KINDNESS

NOTES

GRATITUDE WEEKLY PLANNER

Week of: _____

GRATITUDE goals

TO-DO

	Monday	Tuesday	Wednesday	Thursday	Friday	Saturday	Sunday
ACTIVITIES							
FOCUS							
GRATITUDE							

REFLECTIONS

EXCITED FOR	POSITIVE THOUGHT	KINDNESS

NOTES

GRATITUDE WEEKLY PLANNER

Week of: _____

GRATITUDE *goals*

	Monday	Tuesday	Wednesday	Thursday	Friday	Saturday	Sunday
ACTIVITIES							
FOCUS							
GRATITUDE							

TO-DO

REFLECTIONS

EXCITED FOR	POSITIVE THOUGHT	KINDNESS

NOTES

GRATITUDE WEEKLY PLANNER

Week of: _____

GRATITUDE goals

_____
_____
_____
_____
_____

TO-DO

_____
_____
_____
_____
_____
_____

	Monday	*Tuesday*	*Wednesday*	*Thursday*	*Friday*	*Saturday*	*Sunday*
ACTIVITIES							
FOCUS							
GRATITUDE							

REFLECTIONS

EXCITED FOR	POSITIVE THOUGHT	KINDNESS

NOTES

_____
_____
_____
_____
_____

GRATITUDE WEEKLY PLANNER

Week of: _____

GRATITUDE goals

TO-DO

	Monday	Tuesday	Wednesday	Thursday	Friday	Saturday	Sunday
ACTIVITIES							
FOCUS							
GRATITUDE							

REFLECTIONS

EXCITED FOR	POSITIVE THOUGHT	KINDNESS

NOTES

GRATITUDE WEEKLY PLANNER

Week of: _____

GRATITUDE *goals*

_____
_____
_____
_____
_____

TO-DO

_____
_____
_____
_____
_____
_____
_____

	Monday	Tuesday	Wednesday	Thursday	Friday	Saturday	Sunday
ACTIVITIES							
FOCUS							
GRATITUDE							

REFLECTIONS

EXCITED FOR	POSITIVE THOUGHT	KINDNESS

NOTES

_____
_____
_____
_____
_____

GRATITUDE WEEKLY PLANNER

Week of: _____

GRATITUDE goals

TO-DO

	Monday	*Tuesday*	*Wednesday*	*Thursday*	*Friday*	*Saturday*	*Sunday*
ACTIVITIES							
FOCUS							
GRATITUDE							

REFLECTIONS

EXCITED FOR	POSITIVE THOUGHT	KINDNESS

NOTES

GRATITUDE WEEKLY PLANNER

Week of: _____

GRATITUDE goals

TO-DO

Monday	Tuesday	Wednesday	Thursday	Friday	Saturday	Sunday

ACTIVITIES

FOCUS

GRATITUDE

REFLECTIONS

EXCITED FOR	POSITIVE THOUGHT	KINDNESS

NOTES

GRATITUDE WEEKLY PLANNER

Week of: _____

GRATITUDE *goals*

_____
_____
_____
_____
_____
_____

TO-DO

_____
_____
_____
_____
_____
_____
_____

	Monday	*Tuesday*	*Wednesday*	*Thursday*	*Friday*	*Saturday*	*Sunday*
ACTIVITIES							
FOCUS							
GRATITUDE							

REFLECTIONS

EXCITED FOR	POSITIVE THOUGHT	KINDNESS

NOTES

_____
_____
_____
_____
_____

GRATITUDE WEEKLY PLANNER

Week of: _____

GRATITUDE goals

TO-DO

	Monday	Tuesday	Wednesday	Thursday	Friday	Saturday	Sunday
ACTIVITIES							
FOCUS							
GRATITUDE							

REFLECTIONS

EXCITED FOR	POSITIVE THOUGHT	KINDNESS

NOTES

GRATITUDE WEEKLY PLANNER

Week of: _____

GRATITUDE *goals*

_____
_____
_____
_____
_____
_____

TO-DO

_____
_____
_____
_____
_____
_____

	Monday	Tuesday	Wednesday	Thursday	Friday	Saturday	Sunday
ACTIVITIES							
FOCUS							
GRATITUDE							

REFLECTIONS

EXCITED FOR	POSITIVE THOUGHT	KINDNESS

NOTES

_____
_____
_____
_____
_____

GRATITUDE WEEKLY PLANNER

Week of: _____

GRATITUDE *goals*

Monday | Tuesday | Wednesday | Thursday | Friday | Saturday | Sunday

ACTIVITIES

FOCUS

TO-DO

GRATITUDE

REFLECTIONS

EXCITED FOR | POSITIVE THOUGHT | KINDNESS

NOTES

GRATITUDE WEEKLY PLANNER

Week of: _____

GRATITUDE *goals*

_____
_____
_____
_____
_____

TO-DO

_____
_____
_____
_____
_____

	Monday	*Tuesday*	*Wednesday*	*Thursday*	*Friday*	*Saturday*	*Sunday*
ACTIVITIES							
FOCUS							
GRATITUDE							

REFLECTIONS

EXCITED FOR	POSITIVE THOUGHT	KINDNESS

NOTES

_____
_____
_____
_____
_____

GRATITUDE WEEKLY PLANNER

Week of: _____

GRATITUDE goals

TO-DO

	Monday	Tuesday	Wednesday	Thursday	Friday	Saturday	Sunday
ACTIVITIES							
FOCUS							
GRATITUDE							

REFLECTIONS

EXCITED FOR	POSITIVE THOUGHT	KINDNESS

NOTES

GRATITUDE WEEKLY PLANNER

Week of: _____

GRATITUDE goals

TO-DO

	Monday	Tuesday	Wednesday	Thursday	Friday	Saturday	Sunday
ACTIVITIES							
FOCUS							
GRATITUDE							

REFLECTIONS

EXCITED FOR	POSITIVE THOUGHT	KINDNESS

NOTES

GRATITUDE WEEKLY PLANNER

Week of: _____

GRATITUDE goals

TO-DO

	Monday	Tuesday	Wednesday	Thursday	Friday	Saturday	Sunday
ACTIVITIES							
FOCUS							
GRATITUDE							

REFLECTIONS

EXCITED FOR	POSITIVE THOUGHT	KINDNESS

NOTES

GRATITUDE WEEKLY PLANNER

Week of: _____

GRATITUDE *goals*

_____
_____
_____
_____
_____

TO-DO

_____
_____
_____
_____
_____
_____

	Monday	Tuesday	Wednesday	Thursday	Friday	Saturday	Sunday
ACTIVITIES							
FOCUS							
GRATITUDE							

REFLECTIONS

EXCITED FOR	POSITIVE THOUGHT	KINDNESS

NOTES

_____
_____
_____
_____
_____

GRATITUDE WEEKLY PLANNER

Week of: _____

GRATITUDE goals

_____
_____
_____
_____
_____
_____

TO-DO

_____
_____
_____
_____
_____
_____
_____

	Monday	Tuesday	Wednesday	Thursday	Friday	Saturday	Sunday
ACTIVITIES							
FOCUS							
GRATITUDE							

REFLECTIONS

EXCITED FOR	POSITIVE THOUGHT	KINDNESS

NOTES

_____
_____
_____
_____
_____

GRATITUDE WEEKLY PLANNER

Week of: _____

GRATITUDE goals

_____
_____
_____
_____
_____

TO-DO

_____
_____
_____
_____
_____
_____

	Monday	Tuesday	Wednesday	Thursday	Friday	Saturday	Sunday
ACTIVITIES							
FOCUS							
GRATITUDE							

REFLECTIONS

EXCITED FOR	POSITIVE THOUGHT	KINDNESS

NOTES

_____
_____
_____
_____
_____

GRATITUDE WEEKLY PLANNER

Week of: _____

GRATITUDE goals

TO-DO

	Monday	Tuesday	Wednesday	Thursday	Friday	Saturday	Sunday
ACTIVITIES							
FOCUS							
GRATITUDE							

REFLECTIONS

EXCITED FOR	POSITIVE THOUGHT	KINDNESS

NOTES

GRATITUDE WEEKLY PLANNER

Week of: _____

GRATITUDE goals

_____
_____
_____
_____
_____

TO-DO

_____
_____
_____
_____
_____
_____

	Monday	Tuesday	Wednesday	Thursday	Friday	Saturday	Sunday
ACTIVITIES							
FOCUS							
GRATITUDE							

REFLECTIONS

EXCITED FOR	POSITIVE THOUGHT	KINDNESS

NOTES

_____
_____
_____
_____
_____

GRATITUDE WEEKLY PLANNER

Week of: _____

GRATITUDE goals

TO-DO

	Monday	Tuesday	Wednesday	Thursday	Friday	Saturday	Sunday
ACTIVITIES							
FOCUS							
GRATITUDE							

REFLECTIONS

EXCITED FOR	POSITIVE THOUGHT	KINDNESS

NOTES

GRATITUDE WEEKLY PLANNER

Week of: _____

GRATITUDE goals

- _____
- _____
- _____
- _____
- _____

TO-DO

- _____
- _____
- _____
- _____
- _____

	Monday	Tuesday	Wednesday	Thursday	Friday	Saturday	Sunday
ACTIVITIES							
FOCUS							
GRATITUDE							

REFLECTIONS

EXCITED FOR	POSITIVE THOUGHT	KINDNESS

NOTES

_____
_____
_____
_____

GRATITUDE WEEKLY PLANNER

Week of: _____

GRATITUDE *goals*

_____
_____
_____
_____
_____

TO-DO

_____
_____
_____
_____
_____
_____
_____

	Monday	Tuesday	Wednesday	Thursday	Friday	Saturday	Sunday
ACTIVITIES							
FOCUS							
GRATITUDE							

REFLECTIONS

EXCITED FOR	POSITIVE THOUGHT	KINDNESS

NOTES

_____
_____
_____
_____

GRATITUDE WEEKLY PLANNER

Week of: _____

GRATITUDE goals

_____
_____
_____
_____
_____

TO-DO

_____
_____
_____
_____
_____
_____

	Monday	Tuesday	Wednesday	Thursday	Friday	Saturday	Sunday
ACTIVITIES							
FOCUS							
GRATITUDE							

REFLECTIONS

EXCITED FOR	POSITIVE THOUGHT	KINDNESS

NOTES

_____
_____
_____
_____
_____

GRATITUDE WEEKLY PLANNER

Week of: _____

GRATITUDE goals

_____
_____
_____
_____
_____

TO-DO

_____
_____
_____
_____
_____

	Monday	Tuesday	Wednesday	Thursday	Friday	Saturday	Sunday
ACTIVITIES							
FOCUS							
GRATITUDE							

REFLECTIONS

EXCITED FOR	POSITIVE THOUGHT	KINDNESS

NOTES

_____
_____
_____
_____
_____

GRATITUDE WEEKLY PLANNER

Week of: _____

GRATITUDE *goals*

TO-DO

	Monday	Tuesday	Wednesday	Thursday	Friday	Saturday	Sunday
ACTIVITIES							
FOCUS							
GRATITUDE							

REFLECTIONS

EXCITED FOR	POSITIVE THOUGHT	KINDNESS

NOTES

GRATITUDE WEEKLY PLANNER

Week of: _____

GRATITUDE goals

TO-DO

	Monday	Tuesday	Wednesday	Thursday	Friday	Saturday	Sunday
ACTIVITIES							
FOCUS							
GRATITUDE							

REFLECTIONS

EXCITED FOR	POSITIVE THOUGHT	KINDNESS

NOTES

GRATITUDE WEEKLY PLANNER

Week of: _____

GRATITUDE *goals*

_____
_____
_____
_____
_____
_____

TO-DO

_____
_____
_____
_____
_____
_____

	Monday	Tuesday	Wednesday	Thursday	Friday	Saturday	Sunday
ACTIVITIES							
FOCUS							
GRATITUDE							

REFLECTIONS

EXCITED FOR	POSITIVE THOUGHT	KINDNESS

NOTES

_____
_____
_____
_____
_____

GRATITUDE WEEKLY PLANNER

Week of: _____

GRATITUDE *goals*

_____
_____
_____
_____
_____

TO-DO

_____
_____
_____
_____
_____
_____

	Monday	*Tuesday*	*Wednesday*	*Thursday*	*Friday*	*Saturday*	*Sunday*
ACTIVITIES							
FOCUS							
GRATITUDE							

REFLECTIONS

EXCITED FOR	POSITIVE THOUGHT	KINDNESS

NOTES

_____
_____
_____
_____
_____

GRATITUDE WEEKLY PLANNER

Week of: _____

GRATITUDE goals

TO-DO

	Monday	Tuesday	Wednesday	Thursday	Friday	Saturday	Sunday
ACTIVITIES							
FOCUS							
GRATITUDE							

REFLECTIONS

EXCITED FOR	POSITIVE THOUGHT	KINDNESS

NOTES